AYURVEDIC HEALING PRACTICES

A Comprehensive Guide To Ayurvedic Healing For Digestive Harmony, Musculoskeletal Vitality, Respiratory Well-Being, Radiant Skin, Women's Health, And Men's Vitality

WILFREDO CARSON

INTRODUCTION

Ayurveda, also known as the "science of life," is an ancient method of treatment with profound roots in India's cultural and spiritual traditions.

This holistic approach to healthcare assumes a thorough awareness of the interdependence of the body, mind, and spirit. In this exploration, we will dig into the multifaceted world of Ayurveda, studying its historical evolution, underlying philosophy, and the subtle principles that underlie its medicinal techniques.

1.1 Overview of Ayurveda

Ayurveda is a traditional medical system that has been practiced for thousands of years, making it one of the world's oldest. The phrase "Ayurveda" comes from the Sanskrit words "Ayur" (life) and "Veda" (knowledge or science). This encapsulates the core of Ayurveda, which attempts to provide a thorough understanding of life and its many facets. Unlike traditional medicine, Ayurveda aims to restore balance and harmony within the individual by addressing the core causes of ailments rather than simply treating symptoms.

Ayurveda's key concepts are inextricably linked to the concept of the doshas - Vata, Pitta, and Kapha. These doshas reflect the elemental forces that exist in the body, each of which is accountable for a distinct physiological or psychological function. The balance or imbalance of these doshas determines a person's distinct constitution or Prakriti. Understanding one's Prakriti is important in Ayurveda since it serves as the foundation for tailored health advice such as nutrition, lifestyle, and therapeutic interventions.

1.2 Historical Background and Evolution:

Ayurveda has its roots in the Vedas, which are ancient Indian scriptures, particularly the Rigveda and Atharvaveda. These nearly 5,000-year-old texts include hymns and lyrics that describe Ayurvedic concepts and applications in health maintenance and disease prevention. The accumulation of Ayurvedic knowledge is frequently assigned to the sage Charaka, who wrote the Charaka Samhita, one of the fundamental texts of Ayurveda.

Ayurveda evolved into a comprehensive system that incorporated diverse disciplines such as philosophy, spirituality, and natural healing. Ayurvedic teachings extended throughout the Indian subcontinent, affecting various traditional medical systems in nearby regions. Despite enduring hurdles and periods of decline, Ayurveda has endured throughout history, with increasing interest and acknowledgment in modern times as a significant alternative and supplementary treatment system.

1.3 Philosophy of Ayurveda:

Ayurveda is based on a deep philosophical understanding of the universe, human existence, and the interconnection of all living entities. Ayurvedic philosophy is based on the Panchamahabhutas or the five fundamental elements: earth (Prithvi), water (Jala), fire (Agni), air (Vayu), and ether (Akasha).

These elements unite to produce the three doshas, which represent the dynamic and ever-changing nature of life.

Ayurvedic philosophy is based on the notion that each human is a unique microcosm of the world, with an inherent balance of doshas that determines their physical and mental qualities. This distinct constitution, or Prakriti, determines a person's vulnerability to sickness, preferences, and responses to diverse stimuli. Ayurveda also recognizes the impact of seasons, time of day, and life stages on health and well-being.

Ayurveda's conceptual foundation extends beyond the physical domain, recognizing the close relationship between the body, mind, and spirit. Ayurveda believes that the mind has an important role in both health and sickness. Emotions, beliefs, and mental habits are all important aspects of understanding and treating bodily imbalances. This holistic approach emphasizes the significance of mental and emotional well-being in attaining overall health.

Finally, Ayurveda represents a timeless and holistic approach to healing that extends beyond the mere relief of symptoms.

Its concepts are profoundly entrenched in ancient wisdom, having evolved over millennia to provide a complete understanding of life, health, and the world. As we investigate the fundamentals of Ayurveda, including its overview, historical foundations, and philosophy, we gain insight into a profound system that continues to inspire and assist people on their path to well-being.

CHAPTER 1
FUNDAMENTALS OF AYURVEDA

Ayurveda, an ancient Indian medical system, is based on a deep awareness of nature's interdependence with the human body and psyche. Ayurveda is founded on the concepts of the Pancha Mahabhutas, or the Five Elements, which serve as the universe's essential building blocks. These elements, Earth (Prithvi), Water (Jala), Fire (Agni), Air (Vayu), and Ether (Akasha), are thought to combine in varying quantities to generate the three Doshas: Vata, Pitta, and Kapha. According to Ayurvedic philosophy, maintaining total health and well-being requires a delicate balance of these components and Doshas.

1.1 Five Elements (Pancha Mahabhutas).

Pancha Mahabhutas is the core framework of Ayurveda. Earth, which represents stability and solidity, is linked to the physical structure of the body. Water, which symbolizes fluidity, is linked to biological fluids and their control. Fire, which represents change, governs metabolic processes and digestion. Air, which represents mobility and movement, affects functions such as circulation and breathing. Ether, the most subtle of the elements, represents space and is associated with internal body regions such as hollow organs and channels. The balance and interaction of these factors are thought to determine an individual's constitution, which in turn affects health.

1.1.1 Earth (Prithvi).

In Ayurveda, Earth, or Prithvi, is more than just a physical thing; it also represents stability, hardness, and structure. It is linked to the bones, muscles, and tissues in the human body. When Prithvi is balanced, it provides strength, endurance, and a sense of stability. However, an excess of the Earth element might cause heaviness, lethargy, or stiffness, whilst a shortage can cause weakness and instability. Ayurvedic techniques emphasize balancing the Earth element through food choices, lifestyle changes, and particular therapies to maintain a healthy and strong physical basis.

1.1.2 Water (jala)

In Ayurveda, Jala (water) represents fluidity, cohesiveness, and flexibility. This element governs body fluids like blood, lymph, and mucus. The balance of Jala promotes adequate hydration, joint lubrication, and smooth circulation. An imbalance might lead to diseases like excessive phlegm or dehydration. Ayurvedic remedies for Water element imbalance include dietary changes, herbal formulations, and therapies that promote fluid balance and cleansing, ultimately improving general health and vigor.

1.1.3 Agni (Fire)

Agni, the Fire element in Ayurveda, symbolizes transformation, digestion, and metabolism. This element is essential for the digestion and absorption of nutrients from meals.

A balanced Agni promotes effective digestion, energy production, and mental clarity. On the contrary, an exacerbated Fire element may cause hyperacidity, inflammation, or excessive heat in the body. Dietary changes, medicinal formulations, and lifestyle habits that promote healthy digestive and metabolic functions are all examples of Ayurvedic therapies for preserving Agni homeostasis.

1.1.4 Air (vayu)

Vayu, or air, represents movement, circulation, and transit within the body. It controls breathing, blood circulation, and nerve impulses. Balanced Vayu promotes smooth body functions and mental agility. However, an excess of the Air element can cause symptoms such as gas, bloating, or worry, whilst a shortage can cause stagnation and sluggishness.

Ayurvedic remedies to Vayu imbalance include nutritional suggestions, therapeutic breathwork, and circulation and mobility-enhancing techniques.

1.1.5 Ether (akasha)

Ether, the most delicate element in Ayurveda, symbolizes spaciousness and expansiveness.

It is connected with internal bodily compartments, such as the respiratory and digestive tracts. Ether serves as a container for the other elements and is necessary for the movement of energy. Imbalances in Ether can cause communication problems, such as speech difficulties or trouble expressing oneself. Ayurvedic remedies to harmonize

Ether include techniques such as meditation, sound therapy, and lifestyle changes that promote a sense of spaciousness and clarity in the individual.

1.2 Tridosha Theory.

The Tridosha theory is central to Ayurvedic philosophy, positing that the Five Elements combine to form three essential bioenergetic forces or Doshas: Vata, Pitta, and Kapha. These Doshas regulate different physiological and psychological activities in the body and mind, and their balance is critical for overall wellness.

1.2.1 Vata

Vata, which consists of Air and Ether elements, is connected with mobility, change, and innovation. It regulates functions like respiration, circulation, and nervous system functioning. In a balanced state, Vata encourages flexibility, energy, and fast thinking.

However, an exacerbated Vata can cause anxiety, sleeplessness, and digestive problems. Ayurvedic Vata balancing activities include grounding techniques, nourishing foods, and consistent lifestyle patterns that promote stability and warmth.

1.2.2 Pitta.

Pitta, derived from the Fire and Water elements, represents transformation, digestion, and metabolic processes. It controls activities such as digestion, food absorption, and temperature regulation. A balanced Pitta promotes a powerful digestive fire, a clear mind, and glowing skin. Pitta imbalances can appear as irritation, acidity, or inflammation.

Ayurvedic tactics for calming Pitta include cooling meals, stress management, and activities that foster a calm and composed frame of mind.

1.2.3 Kapha.

Kapha, taken from the Earth and Water elements, represents construction, stability, and lubrication. It regulates physiological fluids, immunological responses, and tissue integrity. A balanced Kapha promotes strength, endurance, and emotional stability. Imbalances in Kapha can cause tiredness, congestion, and weight gain. Ayurvedic ways to balance Kapha include stimulating activities, light and warm diets, and practices that encourage movement and invigoration.

1.3 Prakriti(Constitution)

In Ayurveda, each individual is thought to have a distinct blend of the three Doshas, known as their Prakriti or constitution. Prakriti is determined from conception and remains largely steady throughout one's lifetime. Understanding one's Prakriti is critical in Ayurveda since it leads to personalized health advice such as dietary choices, lifestyle habits, and therapeutic interventions. There are seven different Prakriti combinations, each indicating a distinct Vata, Pitta, or Kapha dominance, or a combination of the three. Tailoring health measures based on an individual's Prakriti enables targeted and effective approaches to maintaining balance and preventing imbalances that can lead to illness.

1.4 Dosha Imbalance and Health.

Ayurveda emphasizes the dynamic nature of health and the importance of balancing the Doshas for total well-being. Imbalances in the Doshas can result from a variety of variables, including diet, lifestyle, environmental effects, and emotional stress. When a Dosha is inflamed or decreased beyond its natural proportion, it can cause physical or mental health problems. Ayurvedic diagnostics entail determining the Dosha imbalance through a thorough evaluation of symptoms, pulse reading, and other observational techniques. Once the imbalance is discovered, tailored treatment plans are developed to restore harmony by targeting the underlying cause rather than just treating the symptoms. Ayurveda's holistic approach defines health as a condition of harmony in the body, mind, and spirit, emphasizing preventive actions and lifestyle changes to sustain optimal well-being.

CHAPTER 2
AYURVEDIC DIAGNOSIS

Ayurveda, an ancient system of medicine that originated in India, emphasizes comprehensive well-being by treating the body, mind, and spirit as linked. Ayurvedic diagnosis is an important component of this holistic approach, incorporating a variety of approaches to identify each individual's unique constitution and imbalances. Ayurvedic diagnosis employs a variety of approaches, including pulse diagnosis (Nadi Pariksha), tongue examination (Jivha Pariksha), face reading (Mukha Pariksha), dosha-specific symptoms, and the use of modern diagnostic instruments.

Analyzing the pulse (Nadi Pariksha)

Nadi Pariksha, also known as pulse diagnosis, is a sophisticated Ayurvedic procedure that assesses an individual's entire health and balance. This method involves examining the radial pulse at numerous wrist positions, with each pulse point representing a unique organ or dosha. Ayurvedic practitioners are trained to detect tiny pulse fluctuations that can indicate imbalances in the three doshas (Vata, Pitta, and Kapha). The pulse is checked for rhythm, pace, strength, and depth, which provide information about the person's physical and mental health.

This ancient diagnostic method enables practitioners to detect dosha imbalances before physical symptoms appear, allowing for early intervention and prevention.

Tongue Exam (Jivha Pariksha):

Jivha Pariksha, or tongue examination, is another important aspect of Ayurvedic diagnosis. The tongue is regarded as a mirror that reflects an individual's interior health. Ayurvedic practitioners carefully examine the color, coating, shape, and texture of the tongue to determine the balance of doshas and the presence of poisons or imbalances in various organs. For example, a white coating on the tongue may indicate excessive Kapha, whereas a yellowish tint may indicate severe Pitta.

The tongue's surface and margins contain important information regarding the digestive system, metabolism, and overall health. Understanding these subtle indicators allows Ayurvedic practitioners to create treatment regimens that restore balance and promote optimal health.

Facial Reading (Mukha Pariksha):

Mukha Pariksha, often known as face reading, is a skilled technique in Ayurveda that involves examining facial features and expressions to learn about a person's constitution and current health. Ayurvedic practitioners evaluate different elements of the face, such as the eyes, nose, lips, forehead, and skin texture. Each face feature is related to a distinct dosha, and its qualities can suggest imbalances or predispositions to certain health disorders. A crimson color in the eyes, for example, may indicate excess

Pitta, whereas dry and flaky skin could indicate high Vata. Mukha Pariksha improves the diagnosis process by providing extra visual signals to support findings from other approaches, resulting in a more complete grasp of the individual's constitution.

<u>Dosha-specific symptoms:</u>

According to Ayurveda, each person's physical, mental, and emotional qualities are determined by a unique combination of the three doshas (Vata, Pitta, and Kapha). Dosha-specific symptoms are important in Ayurvedic diagnosis because they help practitioners identify the prevailing doshas and associated imbalances. Vata imbalances might emerge as anxiety, sleeplessness, or digestive problems, whereas Pitta imbalances can cause inflammation, acidity, or irritation.

Kapha imbalances, on the other hand, can manifest as fatigue, weight gain, or respiratory problems. Ayurvedic practitioners construct treatment programs based on dosha-specific symptoms, including dietary suggestions, lifestyle changes, and herbal medicines, to restore balance and improve general well-being.

Modern Diagnostic Tools in Ayurveda:

While Ayurveda is mainly reliant on ancient diagnostic procedures, the incorporation of modern diagnostic technologies is becoming more common in contemporary Ayurvedic treatments. These tools supplement traditional methods, providing a more complete picture of a person's health status. Blood tests, imaging examinations, and genetic assessments all provide quantifiable information on variables such as blood glucose levels, lipid profiles, and genetic predispositions. Ayurvedic practitioners use this information to fine-tune their diagnoses and create specific treatment programs.

The incorporation of modern diagnostics integrates Ayurveda with current healthcare procedures, encouraging a more collaborative and inclusive approach to overall well-being.

Ayurvedic diagnosis is a rich tapestry of old and modern procedures, each providing unique insights into an individual's constitution and health situation.

Pulse diagnosis, tongue examination, and facial reading give practitioners subtle information, allowing for a more comprehensive comprehension of the patient. Dosha-specific symptoms help tailor treatment strategies and address imbalances at their source. The use of modern diagnostic instruments improves the precision and depth of Ayurvedic diagnosis, connecting old wisdom with modern healthcare procedures. This integrated approach establishes Ayurveda as a holistic system capable of adapting to the changing requirements of people seeking balance and well-being in the modern world.

CHAPTER 3
AYURVEDIC LIFESTYLE PRACTICES

<u>Din Acharya (daily routine):</u>

Din Acharya, or daily routine, is a core idea in Ayurveda that emphasizes the significance of timing daily activities to the natural cycles of the body and environment. The Ayurvedic daily practice is intended to foster balance and harmony within the individual, recognizing the interdependence of the body, mind, and spirit. The day is split into phases, each of which corresponds to a distinct dosha (Vata, Pitta, or Kapha), and activities are organized appropriately. Morning routines frequently include methods such as tongue scraping, oil pulling, and self-massage, which attempt to expel toxins and improve overall health.

Regular meals, proper sleep, and thoughtful activities throughout the day all help to maintain a balanced doshic state, preventing imbalances and encouraging optimal health. Dinacharya is an important part of preventive healthcare in Ayurveda, emphasizing the value of aware and holistic life.

Ritucharya (seasonal routine):

Ritucharya, or seasonal regimen in Ayurveda, acknowledges the dynamic influence of nature on the human body and psyche. This concept highlights the importance of modifying daily routines, diets, and lifestyle choices in response to changing seasons. Ayurveda acknowledges six seasons, each with unique doshic characteristics. Ritucharya advises people on how to adjust their habits to prevent the potential imbalances caused by seasonal shifts.

For example, during the hot and severe summer months (Grishma Ritu), Ayurvedic advice may include cooling foods, drinking, and Pitta dosha-balancing actions. In contrast, in the chilly and damp winter (Shishira Ritu), warming foods, ample relaxation, and activities that balance Kapha dosha may be advised. Ritucharya thus acts as a preventive intervention to align the body with the cyclical pattern of the environment, promoting health and well-being all year.

Sattvik Living:

Sattvic living is a fundamental idea of Ayurveda, emphasizing a lifestyle of purity, balance, and harmony. Sattvic life is derived from the Sanskrit word'sattva,' which implies purity and goodness.

It encourages people to adopt ideas, attitudes, and habits that contribute to a positive and balanced state of being. This idea is inextricably linked to the three gunas (natural states) mentioned in Ayurveda: sattva, rajas, and tamas. Sattvic lifestyle focuses on eating fresh, wholesome foods that nourish the body and soul, promoting mental clarity and spiritual awareness.

It promotes attention, compassion, and self-discipline while avoiding habits that cause negativity or imbalance. Individuals who practice sattvic life seek to align themselves with nature's innate harmony, encouraging overall well-being and a deeper connection to their inner selves.

<u>Yoga & Ayurveda:</u>

The combination of Yoga and Ayurveda is a comprehensive approach to health that considers both physical and mental well-being. Yoga, derived from ancient Indian philosophy, is a technique that uses physical postures (asanas), breath control (pranayama), and meditation to achieve balance and self-realization. The combined approach, which includes Ayurveda, targets an individual's constitution, imbalances, and general health goals. Asanas, or yoga postures, are designed to balance certain doshas while increasing overall flexibility and strength. Pranayama, or breath control, helps regulate the life force energy (prana) in the body, which influences the doshas. Meditation is an essential component that improves mental clarity, reduces stress, and builds a connection with one's inner self. Yoga and Ayurveda work together to help people achieve optimal health by balancing their physical, mental, and spiritual selves.

<u>Asanas:</u>

Yoga's physical postures, or asanas, are critical to the integration of Yoga and Ayurvedic practices. These postures are intended to improve physical health, flexibility, and balance while also altering the subtle energies of the body. Ayurveda prescribes asanas based on an individual's doshic constitution and any underlying imbalances. Individuals with excess Vata may benefit from grounding poses, whilst those with high Pitta may benefit from cooling postures. Regular asana practice is said to increase circulation, digestion, and toxin clearance, all of which contribute to general health. When performed consciously and by Ayurvedic principles, asanas not only promote physical health but also help to balance the doshas and cultivate a harmonious relationship between the body and mind.

Pranayama:

Pranayama, or breath control, is an essential component of the Yoga and Ayurvedic integration. The term 'pranayama' is derived from 'prana' (life force energy) and 'ayama' (control), emphasizing its role in managing subtle energy within the body. Ayurveda stresses the importance of prana in preserving health and avoiding imbalances. Pranayama techniques, such as alternating nostril breathing (Nadi Shodhana) and deep diaphragmatic breathing, are selected based on a person's doshic constitution and health objectives.

Pranayama promotes relaxation, decreases tension, and increases the flow of essential energy throughout the body by controlling the breath. The combined practice of pranayama with Ayurvedic principles contributes to a balanced doshic state, which promotes overall well-being on both a physical and energy level.

<u>Meditation:</u>

Meditation, a major component in the combination of Yoga and Ayurveda, is an effective method for developing mental clarity, emotional balance, and spiritual awareness. Ayurveda recognizes the interdependence of the mind and body, and meditation is said to help harmonize both parts. Meditation is customized to each person's doshic constitution and mental proclivities. Individuals with a Vata dominant may benefit from grounding meditation techniques, whilst those with Pitta imbalances may find comfort in calming practices. Regular meditation is thought to relieve stress, increase self-awareness, and foster inner calm. When paired with Ayurvedic principles, meditation becomes a comprehensive approach to mental well-being, synchronizing the mind with the body's natural rhythms and creating a stronger connection to oneself.

To summarize, Ayurvedic lifestyle practices take a holistic approach to health and well-being, addressing the physical, mental, and spiritual elements of the individual.

Dinacharya and Ritucharya provide instructions for daily and seasonal practices, connecting people to the cyclical rhythm of the environment. Sattvic living emphasizes decisions that promote purity and balance, resulting in overall wellness. The combination of Yoga and Ayurveda emphasizes the interplay of physical postures (asanas), breath control (pranayama), and meditation, providing a comprehensive approach to wellness. Asanas, pranayama, and meditation, when practiced in line with Ayurvedic principles, help to balance the doshas and cultivate overall health. Together, these ideas offer a fundamental foundation for people who want to live in harmony with themselves and the natural environment, encouraging health and vitality on many levels.

pg. 38

CHAPTER 4
AYURVEDIC NUTRITION

Ayurvedic Nutrition is an essential component of Ayurveda, an ancient Indian system of medicine that promotes a comprehensive approach to health and wellness.

It acknowledges the interdependence of the mind, body, and spirit, and sees diet as a tool of achieving internal harmony. Understanding the Six Tastes, or Shad Rasa, is a crucial idea in Ayurvedic nutrition. Each taste is said to have a specific influence on the body and mind, adding to an individual's overall well-being.

The first flavor, Sweet (Madhura), represents sustenance and satisfaction. Sweet-tasting foods are supposed to boost energy, increase strength, and calm nerves.

However, an excessive intake of sugary foods might result in imbalances such as weight gain or sluggishness. The second flavor, sour (amla), is associated with excitement and digestion. Sour foods are thought to improve appetite, digestion, and nutrient absorption. However, excessive consumption of sour foods can lead to acidity and digestive problems.

Salty (Lavana), the third flavor, is linked to hydration and electrolyte balance. Salty meals are supposed to increase hunger, enhance digestion, and maintain adequate fluid balance in the body. On the contrary, eating too many salty meals might cause water retention and high blood pressure. Pungent

(Katu), the fourth taste, is associated with metabolism and cleanliness. Pungent foods are said to improve digestion, circulation, and cleansing. Excessive intake, on the other hand, might cause the body to overheat and aggravate certain illnesses.

Bitter (Tikta), the fifth flavor, is linked to detoxification and purification. Bitter meals are supposed to detoxify the body, purify the blood, and improve liver function. However, eating too many bitter foods might cause an imbalance in the Vata dosha, resulting in dryness and constipation. Astringent (Kashaya), the sixth taste, is associated with absorption and toning. Astringent meals are thought to improve nutrient absorption, tighten tissues, and give a cooling impact. However, excessive use might cause dryness and tightness in the body.

Food as Medicine is a fundamental principle of Ayurvedic Nutrition, which emphasizes the healing benefits of certain foods.

In Ayurveda, each individual is regarded as unique, and food selection is based on one's constitution (Prakriti), the present state of health (Vikriti), and external variables. Foods are classed according to their intrinsic properties and effects on the doshas (Vata, Pitta, and Kapha). Warming foods, such as ginger and cayenne pepper, may be recommended for people with a strong Vata dosha to balance its chilly and dry properties.

Furthermore, Ayurveda understands the value of attentive eating. It implies that the state of mind when eating affects the digestion and assimilation process. Stress, worry, and unpleasant emotions during meals are thought to impede healthy digestion and nutrient absorption. As a result, Ayurvedic practices encourage people to eat in a calm and serene environment, which promotes a happy and relaxed attitude.

Ayurvedic cooking methods play an important role in conserving foods' intrinsic properties and enhancing their nutritional worth. Different cooking methods are recommended depending on the nature of the components and the desired doshic balance. For example, boiling and steaming are moderate cooking methods that help keep the natural flavors and nutrients of the food, making them appropriate for people with Pitta or Kapha imbalances.

Roasting and grilling, on the other hand, are thought to be better at balancing excess Kapha since they give the dish a warming feel.

The type of cooking oil is also an important concern in Ayurvedic cookery, with different oils advised for each dosha. Cooling oils, such as coconut or olive oil, may be chosen by Pitta folks, whilst warming oils, such as mustard or sesame oil, are indicated for Vata balance.

Dietary Guidelines for Dosha Balance improves Ayurvedic nutrition by making individualized suggestions to individuals based on their prevalent dosha or doshic imbalances. Ayurveda distinguishes three basic doshas: Vata, Pitta, and Kapha, each with distinct attributes and characteristics.

The prevalent dosha at the time of conception determines a person's constitution, known as

Prakriti. Dietary guidelines are intended to balance the doshas and sustain internal harmony.

Ayurvedic advice for people with a prominent Vata dosha may include warm, grounding foods such as cooked grains, root vegetables, and nutritious soups.

To balance Pitta dosha, people should eat cooling and hydrating foods like cucumbers, mint, and sweet fruits. Kapha people may benefit from lighter, warmer, and stimulating foods like spicy soups, bitter greens, and astringent fruits.

Furthermore, Ayurvedic food instructions take into account seasonal fluctuations and the effects of external influences on the doshas. For example, during the chilly winter months, people with Vata imbalances may be urged to eat warm, nourishing foods to counteract the cold and dry weather.

Finally, Ayurvedic Nutrition includes a thorough study of the Six Tastes, the medicinal significance of food, culinary techniques, and tailored dietary suggestions based on dosha balance. It reflects Ayurveda's holistic approach, which emphasizes the interdependence of physical, mental, and spiritual well-being. Individuals who incorporate these concepts into their daily lives can strive for balance, harmony, and optimal health through Ayurvedic therapeutic practices.

CHAPTER 5
AYURVEDIC HERBAL MEDICINE

A Brief Overview of Ayurvedic Herbs

Ayurvedic Herbal Medicine, a key component of Ayurveda, is a holistic and traditional treatment approach that has been practiced for thousands of years. Ayurveda, which is based on ancient Indian wisdom, emphasizes the balance of mind, body, and spirit to promote overall health. Herbal remedies are central to Ayurvedic treatments and serve as the foundation for therapeutic interventions.

The technique is customized, taking into account each individual's unique constitution, known as doshas (Vata, Pitta, and Kapha), and aims to restore balance using the innate healing powers of specific plants.

<u>Common Ayurvedic herbs:</u>

A wide range of botanicals are used in Ayurvedic Herbal Medicine to provide therapeutic advantages. Each plant has unique properties and is given depending on its compatibility with a person's constitution and the nature of the illness. Among the regularly used herbs, Ashwagandha stands out for its adaptogenic characteristics, which improve the body's ability to tolerate stress. Turmeric, known for its anti-inflammatory and antioxidant properties, is an important ingredient in many Ayurvedic formulas. Triphala, a combination of three fruits, is a powerful digestive tonic, while Neem is known for its antibacterial properties. Tulsi, or Holy Basil, is another well-known herb for its immune-boosting and stress-relieving properties.

<u>Ayurvedic formulations:</u>

Ayurvedic formulations combine multiple herbs to achieve synergistic effects that improve therapeutic outcomes.

These formulations are methodically developed to address specific health conditions, taking into account the individual's dosha, the nature of the disease, and the desired therapeutic results. The synergy of herbs in preparation is said to have a holistic effect, addressing the underlying cause of the imbalance rather than only treating symptoms. Formulations are frequently made in the form of powders, decoctions, or oils that are customized to the individual's constitution and the condition being treated. Ayurvedic practitioners prescribe these compositions with a thorough grasp of the herbs' characteristics and interactions.

<u>Ayurveda Pharmacy:</u>

The notion of Ayurvedic Pharmacy includes the sourcing, processing, and production of herbal medications by Ayurvedic guidelines. The quality of the herbs, extraction procedures, and preparation techniques all play an important part in determining the efficacy of the finished product. Traditional procedures, such as Ayurvedic pharmacopeia, oversee the production of herbal medications, assuring consistency and authenticity. The pharmacy procedure includes selecting the right herbs, washing and processing them precisely, and mixing them in the proper amounts to make effective formulations. Quality control measures are implemented to ensure that the medications are pure and safe while adhering to Ayurvedic principles of holistic health.

Finally, Ayurvedic Herbal Medicine exemplifies Ayurveda's long legacy by emphasizing tailored care and comprehensive healing. The deep knowledge of plants, their synergy, and the precise manufacture of formulations in Ayurvedic Pharmacy all contribute to the ancient medical system's efficiency. As Ayurveda obtains global awareness, the incorporation of Ayurvedic Herbal Medicine into mainstream healthcare demonstrates a growing appreciation for the benefits of holistic and customized approaches to well-being.

CHAPTER 6
AYURVEDIC THERAPIES

The ancient Indian medical method known as Ayurveda emphasizes holistic therapy, which involves harmonizing the mind, body, and spirit. Ayurvedic medicines play an important role in establishing this balance by addressing both the symptoms and the underlying causes of ailments. Panchakarma, a comprehensive detoxification and rejuvenation process, is a pillar of Ayurveda therapy.

6.1 Panchakarma.

Panchakarma is a Sanskrit phrase that means "five actions" and refers to a set of therapeutic operations aimed at purifying the body. These treatments are intended to clear toxins, restore equilibrium to the doshas (Vata, Pitta, and

Kapha), and enhance overall health. Panchakarma has five major procedures: Vamana (emesis), Virechana (purgation), Basti (enema), Nasya (nasal administration), and Raktamokshana (bloodletting).

6.1.1 Vamana

Vamana, or therapeutic vomiting, is a Panchakarma treatment that specifically targets the Kapha dosha. This procedure involves administering emetic drugs to cause controlled vomiting, which eliminates excess Kapha-related toxins from the upper respiratory tract and stomach. Vamana is very effective for bronchial asthma, allergies, and skin diseases caused by aggravated Kapha.

6.1.2 Virechana.

Virechana, the second Panchakarma process, targets the Pitta dosha and entails regulated purgation. Patients are given purgatives to cleanse their digestive tract, liver, and gallbladder, eliminating excess Pitta-related toxins. This therapy is widely used to treat illnesses such as liver ailments, jaundice, and skin diseases caused by exacerbated Pitta.

6.1.3 Basta

Basti, or therapeutic enema, is a Panchakarma treatment that targets Vata dosha imbalances. It entails administering therapeutic chemicals into the rectum to cleanse the colon and nourish the tissues. Basti is very useful for illnesses such as constipation, lower back discomfort, and neurological disorders caused by exacerbated Vata.

6.1.4 Nasya.

Nasya, a nasal administration therapy in Panchakarma, aims to balance the Kapha and

Vata doshas. Medicated oils or powders are delivered into the nasal passages to relieve sinus congestion, improve respiratory function, and increase mental clarity. Nasya is frequently used to treat headaches, sinusitis, and neurological diseases associated with Kapha and Vata imbalances.

6.1.5 Rakatamokshana

Raktamokshana, the fifth Panchakarma process, is the therapeutic evacuation of blood to cleanse impurities and balance Pitta dosha. This traditional bloodletting procedure is rarely utilized in modern Ayurvedic practice, but it may be explored in select circumstances, such as skin problems and conditions linked to high Pitta levels.

6.2 Ayurvedic Massage (Abhyanga).

Ayurvedic massage, also known as Abhyanga, is an essential component of Ayurvedic self-care and therapeutic therapies. This massage involves applying warm, medicinal oils to the entire body, which promotes relaxation, better circulation, and toxin discharge. Abhyanga is essential for balancing the doshas, moisturizing the skin, and improving overall health. The selection of oils is frequently tailored to the individual's constitution and unique health conditions, giving Abhyanga a personalized and refreshing experience.

6.3 Mara Therapy

Marma treatment is a distinct branch of Ayurvedic medicine that focuses on critical energy centers throughout the body known as marma points. These spots are regarded as intersections of the body's life force, and manipulating them is thought to impact the flow of energy and facilitate healing. Marma treatment uses moderate pressure, massage, and energy work to balance the doshas, relieve pain, and boost overall well-being. Practitioners meticulously examine each individual's constitution and specific health challenges before tailoring marma therapy sessions for the best results.

6.4 Sound and Colour Therapy in Ayurveda

Sound and color therapy are essential components of Ayurvedic medicine, which uses the vibrational capabilities of sound and the therapeutic properties of colors to restore balance and harmony to the mind and body. Sound therapy, also known as Nada Yoga, is the application of certain sounds, chants, and mantras to alter the doshas and produce a therapeutic resonance within the body. Similarly, color treatment, also known as chromotherapy, uses visual stimulation with certain hues to elicit physiological and psychological reactions.

Ayurveda associates each dosha with unique colors and sounds, and therapeutic approaches are chosen based on an individual's doshic constitution. For example, the relaxing influence of blue light may be recommended for Pitta-related disorders, whilst warm and anchoring tones may aid Vata imbalances. Sound and color therapy are used with other Ayurvedic methods to improve overall health, alleviate stress, and promote balance.

Finally, Ayurvedic therapies are a diverse set of holistic healing approaches that strive to balance the mind, body, and spirit. Panchakarma, Ayurvedic massage (Abhyanga), Marma treatment, and sound and color therapy are all part of this ancient system of medicine, with each having its approach to addressing imbalances and promoting maximum health. These therapies aim not merely to relieve symptoms, but also to restore the doshas' underlying balance, promoting long-term well-being and vigor. As people seek more holistic approaches to health and wellness, Ayurvedic therapies continue to play an important role in providing comprehensive and customized healing experiences.

CHAPTER 7
AYURVEDA AND THE MIND~ BODY CONNECTION

Ayurveda, an ancient school of medicine that originated in India, emphasizes the mind-body link. This holistic approach sees a person as a complex interaction of physical, mental, and spiritual aspects. The notion of Ayurvedic Psychology encompasses a knowledge of psychological well-being in the context of Ayurvedic treatment procedures.

This paradigm goes beyond simply treating physical symptoms; it investigates the complex balance between the mind and body, acknowledging the tremendous impact of mental states on total health.

Ayurvedic Psychology, as a fundamental principle, holds that the mind is a powerful force that influences the body's homeostasis.

It is based on the premise that mental and emotional states, such as stress, worry, or happiness, can manifest physically and affect many physiological activities. Ayurveda divides the mind into three key qualities called Gunas: Sattva, Rajas, and Tamas.

Sattva depicts purity, clarity, and harmony, whereas Rajas represents activity, restlessness, and passion. Tamas is related to inactivity, dullness, and sluggishness. Balancing these Gunas is critical for mental health, as imbalances can lead to diseases.

Managing stress is a critical component of Ayurvedic therapy, which prompts us to investigate how Ayurveda approaches stress management.

Stress has become an unavoidable aspect of modern life, and its negative consequences on health are well known. However, Ayurveda offers a more subtle and complete approach to stress management. It recognizes that stress is a complex interplay of psychological, physiological, and environmental elements, rather than a purely mental issue.

Stress is viewed in Ayurveda as an imbalance in the Doshas, the basic forces that control the body.

Ayurvedic stress treatment entails determining an individual's unique constitution, or Prakriti, and evaluating the Dosha imbalances that contribute to stress.

The Vata, Pitta, and Kapha Doshas all play important roles in stress responses.

For example, an exacerbated Vata may cause anxiety and restlessness, whereas an imbalanced Pitta might cause impatience and rage. Kapha imbalance can cause fatigue and a sense of heaviness. Ayurvedic stress management therapies include dietary adjustments, lifestyle changes, herbal remedies, and yoga and meditation activities that are customized to individual Dosha imbalances.

Ayurveda defines mental and emotional well-being as more than just the absence of stress.

It encompasses a state of equilibrium in which the intellect is clear, emotions are balanced, and the individual feels content.

Ayurvedic concepts for mental and emotional well-being center on cultivating Sattva, a trait linked with purity and harmony. Sattvic foods are fresh, clean, and pure, and are said to nourish the intellect and foster emotional harmony. Furthermore, engaging in activities that promote a healthy state of mind, such as meditation and mindfulness techniques, is essential to Ayurvedic approaches to mental health.

Ayurvedic psychology recognizes the influence of environmental variables on mental health, such as the environment, relationships, and lifestyle. Unhealthy relationships, exposure to chemicals, and an unbalanced schedule can all lead to mental and emotional distress. As a result, Ayurveda urges people to create a supportive environment and adopt lifestyle behaviors that are compatible with their Prakriti and Dosha balance. This individualized approach acknowledges each individual's uniqueness and emphasizes the value of tailored interventions for mental health.

Finally, Ayurveda's examination of the mind-body connection demonstrates its comprehensive and customized approach to health. Ayurvedic Psychology investigates the complex connection between the mind and body, acknowledging the deep influence of mental states on total well-being.

Ayurvedic stress management requires a thorough understanding of an individual's constitution and Dosha imbalances, with interventions ranging from dietary changes to mindfulness activities. The quest for mental and emotional well-being in Ayurveda goes beyond stress management, emphasizing the cultivation of Sattva and customized lifestyle routines to promote balance. Overall, Ayurvedic treatment practices provide a thorough awareness of the interconnection of mental, bodily, and spiritual components, hence providing a comprehensive road map to well-being.

CHAPTER 8
AYURVEDA FOR SPECIFIC HEALTH CONDITIONS

Ayurveda, an ancient method of holistic therapy that originated in India, provides a comprehensive approach to health and wellness. It emphasizes the balance of mind, body, and spirit while taking into account individual constitutions, or doshas, which include Vata, Pitta, and Kapha. Ayurvedic treatment procedures are adapted to individual health issues, to restore internal harmony and balance. In this examination, we will look at Ayurvedic approaches to a variety of health issues, including digestive diseases, joint and musculoskeletal health, respiratory conditions, skin disorders, women's health, and men's health.

Digestive issues are a serious health challenge for many people, often resulting in discomfort and poor overall well-being. Ayurveda recognizes the value of a well-balanced digestive tract for overall health. According to Ayurvedic beliefs, the digestive fire, or Agni, is essential for nutritional assimilation and waste disposal. When Agni is unbalanced, a variety of digestive issues might arise. Ayurvedic treatments for digestive problems include dietary changes, herbal therapies, and lifestyle changes. Digestive herbs like triphala and ginger are often used to improve digestion and relieve symptoms. Furthermore, mindful eating behaviors, such as eating warm, freshly prepared meals and avoiding incompatible food combinations, are key components of Ayurvedic guidelines for digestive health.

Ayurvedic medicine also focuses on joint and musculoskeletal wellness. In Ayurvedic philosophy, an imbalance in the Vata dosha is frequently related to joint and musculoskeletal diseases. The emphasis is on keeping joints properly lubricated and nourished to avoid problems like arthritis. Herbal formulations, external applications such as medicinal oils and poultices, and specific dietary and lifestyle recommendations are all examples of Ayurvedic joint health treatments. Panchakarma, an Ayurvedic detoxification therapy, is also used to get rid of toxins that can cause joint problems. In Ayurveda, it is usual to use anti-inflammatory herbs such as turmeric and Boswellia serrata in the diet to treat joint difficulties.

Respiratory problems, ranging from simple colds to chronic respiratory ailments, are treated using Ayurvedic concepts that emphasize regulating the Kapha dosha. Ayurveda emphasizes the necessity of having clear and unobstructed respiratory airways for overall wellness. Herbal compositions including expectorant and anti-inflammatory herbs like licorice, tulsi, and ginger are frequently prescribed to relieve respiratory problems. Steam inhalation with eucalyptus or mint oils is a traditional method for soothing the respiratory system. Pranayama, a series of breathing exercises, is also recommended to improve lung function and respiratory health. Ayurvedic dietary guidelines for respiratory disorders include limiting mucus-forming foods and integrating warming spices to regulate Kapha.

Ayurveda treats skin diseases holistically, including acne and psoriasis.

The skin is seen to be a reflection of an individual's general health, and dosha imbalances can cause a variety of skin problems. Ayurvedic remedies for skin diseases combine internal and exterior therapies. Internal purification using Panchakarma, dietary changes, and the usage of certain herbs like neem, turmeric, and aloe vera are prominent strategies. External treatments include medicinal oils, herbal pastes, and baths that nourish and revitalize the skin. Ayurvedic practitioners also emphasize the emotional and psychological components of skin health, stressing stress reduction and lifestyle changes to improve skin well-being.

Women's health is a major focus of Ayurveda, which recognizes the distinct physiological and hormonal changes that women experience throughout their lives. Ayurvedic approaches to women's health include understanding and harmonizing the menstrual cycle, promoting fertility, and treating disorders including polycystic ovarian syndrome (PCOS) and menopausal symptoms. Herbal formulations comprising herbs such as Shatavari and ashwagandha are frequently prescribed to promote hormonal balance. Ayurvedic dietary advice for women's health stresses nutritious meals while avoiding processed and inflammatory items. Specific yoga postures and pranayama are recommended as part of a healthy lifestyle.

Similarly, Ayurveda approaches men's health with a focus on their specific constitution and health concerns. Ayurvedic therapies for men's health include maintaining reproductive health, balancing testosterone levels, and treating erectile dysfunction and prostate disorders. Herbs like ashwagandha and gokshura are often used to improve male reproductive health. Dietary guidelines stress the consumption of nutrient-dense meals while avoiding highly processed and spicy foods. Ayurvedic lifestyle advice for men includes regular exercise, stress management techniques, and the development of healthy daily routines to enhance vitality and longevity.

Finally, Ayurveda offers a holistic and tailored approach to treating specific health concerns. Ayurvedic therapeutic procedures seek to restore balance and harmony in the body by taking into account each person's unique constitution and the interaction of doshas. The combination of herbal medicines, dietary changes, lifestyle changes, and therapeutic procedures like Panchakarma demonstrates Ayurveda's complete approach to promoting health and well-being. As an old system with a rich legacy, Ayurveda continues to provide useful insights and practical solutions to modern health issues, emphasizing the interdependence of mind, body, and spirit in the pursuit of optimal health.

CHAPTER 9
INTEGRATING AYURVEDA AND MODERN MEDICINE

Ayurveda, an ancient system of medicine originating in India, has garnered global recognition for its comprehensive approach to health and wellness. Integrating Ayurveda with contemporary medicine, sometimes known as allopathy, has sparked great interest and controversy in the healthcare world. Ayurveda and allopathy are two independent paradigms, each with its own beliefs and procedures. Ayurveda, which has its roots in ancient writings such as the Charaka Samhita and Sushruta Samhita, emphasizes the balance of three doshas (Vata, Pitta, and Kapha) and concentrates on specific treatment programs based on an individual's constitution. On the other hand, allopathy is based on evidence-based treatments, medicinal interventions, and surgical procedures.

<u>Ayurveda and Allopathy.</u>

The confluence of Ayurveda and Allopathy presents both obstacles and opportunities. While Ayurveda and allopathy have fundamentally different conceptual frameworks, there is an increasing recognition of potential synergies between the two systems. Ayurveda's emphasis on preventive healthcare, lifestyle changes, and natural cures is consistent with the current trend toward holistic well-being. Allopathy, with its sophisticated diagnostics and technology solutions, excels in acute care and emergencies. The problem is to bridge the gap between Ayurvedic medicine's customized, nature-based approach and allopathy's standardized, scientifically validated methodologies.

As Ayurveda gains popularity, efforts are being made to develop collaborative approaches that leverage the benefits of both systems. Integrative medicine, which blends Ayurveda and allopathy in complementary ways, is gaining popularity. This approach attempts to provide patients with a comprehensive healthcare experience that tackles the underlying causes of illness while taking advantage of modern medical advances. The collaboration goes beyond treatment and includes research, teaching, and the creation of guidelines to help practitioners negotiate the integration effectively.

Holistic Healthcare Approach

One of the most important components of combining Ayurveda and contemporary medicine is adopting a holistic healthcare approach. Ayurveda, as a comprehensive system, analyzes not just physical symptoms but also mental health, lifestyle, and environmental effects. This contrasts with the reductionist approach commonly associated with allopathy, which focuses on individual symptoms or organ systems. The holistic paradigm promotes a more comprehensive knowledge of health and disease, supporting a patient-centered approach that considers the interdependence of different areas of a person's life.

In the integrated healthcare concept, practitioners from Ayurveda and allopathy work together to develop treatment strategies that combine the best of both worlds. This could include integrating Ayurvedic dietary recommendations, herbal formulations, and lifestyle changes with allopathic drugs and therapies. The goal is to offer patients a comprehensive and tailored strategy that takes into account the complex interaction of physical, mental, and emotional aspects influencing their health.

<u>Case Studies</u>

Examining case studies is an effective way to evaluate the practical implications and effects of merging Ayurveda and modern medicine. These case studies provided insight into the efficacy, obstacles, and possible benefits of collaborative healthcare practices. Researchers and healthcare practitioners are increasingly documenting cases in which patients received both Ayurvedic and allopathic therapies, providing insights into the efficacy of such integrative techniques.

Chronic diseases are a major topic of investigation, as the limitations of conventional allopathic treatments are obvious. Case studies of autoimmune disorders, metabolic syndromes, and lifestyle diseases demonstrate how Ayurvedic principles can supplement modern medical interventions. By studying patient outcomes, researchers hope to find patterns, refine treatment regimens, and add to the expanding body of evidence supporting the merger of Ayurveda and contemporary medicine.

CONCLUSION

The confluence of Ayurveda with modern medicine represents a dynamic and changing frontier in healthcare.

The cohabitation of these two systems provides a rare chance to blend traditional wisdom with cutting-edge scientific breakthroughs, resulting in a more complete and patient-centered approach to healing. The collaboration between Ayurveda and allopathy recognizes each system's strengths, to combine Ayurvedic holistic principles with contemporary medicine's diagnostic and therapeutic skills.

The obstacles to this integration should not be underestimated. Various philosophies, diagnostic techniques, and treatment methodologies necessitate a thorough and informed analysis. However, the potential benefits are significant, ranging from improved preventive care and chronic illness management to a more tailored and long-term healthcare strategy. Ayurveda's holistic approach, with its emphasis on balance and harmony, complements modern medicine's reductionist approach, resulting in a synergy capable of addressing the complexities of human health.

As we move forward, research efforts, joint clinical trials, and multidisciplinary training programs will become increasingly important. Establishing a common platform of communication and understanding between Ayurvedic practitioners and allopathic experts is critical to the success of integrated treatment. This coordinated effort includes education, as future generations of healthcare providers must have a thorough understanding of both systems.

In the grand scheme of healthcare, the merger of Ayurveda and contemporary medicine symbolizes a paradigm change toward a more inclusive, patient-centered approach.

It necessitates a dedication to open-mindedness, scientific rigor, and a common goal for individual and communal well-being. While problems remain, the potential benefits of improved patient outcomes, holistic health promotion, and a more sustainable healthcare system make the journey toward integrated healing practices an appealing and hopeful endeavor.